The BOOK of TAPPING

The BOOK of TAPPING

Emotional Acupressure

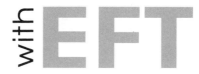

SOPHIE MERLE

Translated by Jon E. Graham

Healing Arts Press

Rochester, Vermont • Toronto, Canada

Healing Arts Press
One Park Street
Rochester, Vermont 05767
www.HealingArtsPress.com

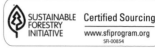

Text stock is SFI certified

Healing Arts Press is a division of Inner Traditions International

Originally published in France under the title *EFT psychologie énergétique: Le livre pour se libérer des blocages et troubles émotionnels* by Éditions Médicis
First U.S. edition published in 2017 by Healing Arts Press

Note to the reader: *This book is intended as an informational guide. The remedies, approaches, and techniques described herein are meant to supplement, and not to be a substitute for, professional medical care or treatment. They should not be used to treat a serious ailment without prior consultation with a qualified health care professional.*

Library of Congress Cataloging-in-Publication Data

Names: Merle, Sophie, author.
Title: The book of tapping : emotional acupressure with EFT / Sophie Merle; translated by Jon E. Graham.
Other titles: EFT Psychologie Énergétique. French
Description: First U.S. edition. | Rochester, Vermont : Healing Arts Press, 2017. | Includes bibliographical references and index.
Identifiers: LCCN 2016041276 (print) | LCCN 2016048867 (e-book) | ISBN 9781620556016 (paperback) | ISBN 9781620556023 (e-book)
Subjects: LCSH: Acupuncture points—Popular works. | Self-help techniques. | BISAC: HEALTH & FITNESS / Acupressure & Acupuncture (see also MEDICAL / Acupuncture). | SELF-HELP / Stress Management. | BODY, MIND & SPIRIT / Healing / Energy (Chi Kung, Reiki, Polarity).
Classification: LCC RM723.A27 M47 2017 (print) | LCC RM723.A27 (e-book) | DDC 615.8/92—dc23
LC record available at https://lccn.loc.gov/2016041276

Printed and bound in the United States by Lake Book Manufacturing, Inc. The text stock is SFI certified. The Sustainable Forestry Initiative® program promotes sustainable forest management.

10 9 8 7 6 5 4 3 2

Text design and layout by Virginia Scott Bowman
This book was typeset in Garamond Premier Pro with Guardi, Helvetica, and Avenir used as display typefaces.

To send correspondence to the author of this book, mail a first-class letter to the author c/o Inner Traditions • Bear & Company, One Park Street, Rochester, VT 05767, and we will forward the communication, or contact the author directly at **www.SophieMerle.com** (website in French).

Contents

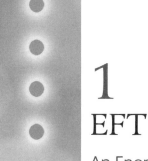

1
EFT

An Energetic Technique for Health
and Material Abundance

The letters "EFT" are commonly used to represent a new treatment procedure, Emotional Freedom Technique, that has been the subject of much talk in recent years. Because its treatment methods are easy to use and produce sensational results, EFT is a fascinating topic.

The central tenet of its theory is that any discontent or disorder in our lives is the result of an imbalance in the energy that flows through our physical bodies. Its main concern is the restoration of harmony using the meridian points of Chinese acupuncture, for which EFT is an emotion-based variation.

EFT is also known as psychological acupuncture, meridian therapy, and, most commonly, Tapping therapy, or simply Tapping. This term refers to the light tapping of meridian points during a treatment session. The term Tapping (capitalized) will be used throughout this book in reference to the EFT protocol, because it is the most convenient expression, while *tapping* (lowercase) refers to the actual hand movement.

The use of the body's meridians to restore physical health has been commonplace in China for an extremely long time. Although it has become more accepted in the West today, it was not used for the treatment of emotional suffering until quite recently. Proponents of EFT believe that such suffering is caused by blockages in the body's energy system, in which each meridian point represents a series of specific emotions (for more information see the section beginning on page 56).

EFT focuses its attention exclusively on removing these energy blockages in order to restore our sense of well-being. The process has been the driving force for some spectacular healings and strongly indicates that negative emotions are due to a disruption in the body's energy system. In many cases, once balance has been restored to the energy flow, negative emotions vanish, thereby also removing the problems that accompanied this imbalance.

THE BIRTH AND DEVELOPMENT OF EFT

EFT emerged from the initial modality of this type, TFT (Thought Field Therapy), which was created in the 1980s by psychiatrist Roger Callahan, a bold pioneer in a new era in the field of psychology. He was the first individual, in both East and West, to use the meridians for healing emotional problems.

However, Dr. Callahan's procedure is extremely complex. It requires a precise diagnosis of the points that need stimulation and calls for them to be stimulated in a particular sequences for each problem, which makes his method impractical without the help of an experienced practitioner. In the 1990s, following an extensive study of TFT, Gary Craig, a nondenominational ordained minister and certified master practitioner in neurolinguistic programming (NLP), figured out how to avoid this difficulty through the practice of EFT, in which the same sequences of point stimulation, more commonly referred to as Tapping, can be used in the treatment of any kind of emotional issue.

EFT's worldwide success is due to its simplicity of use as well as its effectiveness, which is often superior to that of other healing techniques. Numerous health professionals employ it, either by itself or as a supplement to more traditional treatment, and play an active role in its growing popularity by frequently publicizing its effectiveness in promoting rapid healing of critical physical and mental health problems.*

Making it even more appealing, this procedure is simple to master, and although it is best learned from a professional, either in person or via teaching materials, it can be regularly used to control personal health problems without the need of additional help. This is an invaluable option for those who have limited access to professional care.

---

*As of 2016, more than 80 research studies had been published on energy psychology modalities; for details see the Association for Comprehensive Energy Psychology (ACEP) website, which is listed in the resources section of this book.

EFT IN A NUTSHELL

EFT can be summed up as the stimulation of several specific points on the face, upper torso, and hands while the individual concentrates at the same time on a specific difficulty. This should be done until all accompanying negative feelings disappear completely. The biggest challenge lies in determining and then administering the appropriate number of rounds of tapping required to completely uproot and remove these upsetting emotions. Were it not for this, EFT would be so simple that even children could use it by themselves.

A number of psychotherapists incorporate Tapping in their practice and are qualified to teach the proper use of the protocol, and there are numerous online tutorial videos and listings of EFT workshops (see the resources section in the back of the book), but no knowledge of psychology is necessary to make good use of the technique. EFT is the instrument of choice for personal development and will soon make all other methods seem obsolete— especially methods that ask us to use mind control or the power of positive thinking all by itself to curb negative feelings. It is impossible for such approaches to work effectively, as the required state of vigilance is difficult to sustain. Moreover, negative thoughts have an energetic component, and when energy blockages occur, they require physical stimulation of the energy system to dissipate. This somewhat explains why a long walk outdoors can be beneficial in eliminating nonclinical depression.

Nor is it necessary to "believe in" EFT to obtain results. Most people begin the process with great skepticism because its basic concept goes against our ingrained belief systems. But we'd better get used to it, because the era of energetic healing techniques has begun and can only expand rapidly. As Gary Craig likes to say, "We are on the ground floor of a new healing high-rise," and there is no end to the potential for surprises.

EFT'S BENEFITS

Learning the basics of EFT should not take you more than a couple of hours. It will then allow you to do things you thought impossible to accomplish before, such as speaking in public or flying in an airplane without fear. The extent of the ways in which EFT can help us is practically infinite. It makes sense to try it on any problem, even those issues that seem impossible to solve. Some of the common problems EFT can eliminate are:

- **Phobias.** EFT quickly liberates us from the anguish of agoraphobia, claustrophobia, and any other fears or aversions, regardless of how long they have existed or how terrifying they may feel. It also stops panic attacks in their tracks, usually quite quickly.
- **Tragic memories.** The emotional pain of traumatic memories melts away, along with any regret, fear, anger, or guilt they inspire. The past no longer

has a malignant grip on the present. The memories remain, but they have been stripped of their ability to cause pain.

• **Irresistible urges.** EFT is able to rapidly halt any desire at the moment it is first felt. This could be the desire for a cigarette (EFT is especially amazing for a smoker on a long airplane flight), alcohol, drugs, or foods forbidden by a diet. The anxiety behind the need vanishes, as does the need to fight anxiety by ingesting certain substances.

• **Difficult emotions.** Tapping can remove anxiety, discouragement, bitterness, regret, obsession, anger, frustration, resignation, dismay, shame, lack of self-confidence, and stage fright, as well as feelings of abandonment, rejection, jealousy, and so on. EFT can also rapidly soothe the pain of a broken heart.

• **Restrictive beliefs.** EFT neutralizes mental limitations, which can be powerful hindrances to achieving ambitions in any aspect of life: professional, academic, sports, financial, or relational. It is the ideal procedure for improving performance in any domain.

• **Illness and physical suffering.** The contribution of EFT in this domain is remarkable, with a very impressive list of case studies (see the ACEP website). It is recommended as a potent supplement to traditional treatments for any kind of physical ailment, and it improves the effect of medications.

It can also be used to treat weight problems and insomnia, and it dispels nightmares as well.

EVERYTHING IS ENERGY

It is commonly believed in the Western world that matter and energy are entirely separate things. However, to understand how EFT works, it is important to recognize that we live in a world comprised of a single energy. It is a primordial force that imagines, engenders, and connects everything that exists in creation.

On the underlying level of our reality, this single energy mass is continually in movement. It is only a vibrational diversity that makes things appear to be distinct from each other, while time and space appear to separate things and events.

Our circumstances in life are purely energetic in nature, as are the beliefs, thoughts, and emotions that create these circumstances. Because of this, our problems are of a purely energetic nature as well. They arise from a vibratory dissonance between what we already have in life and what we would prefer to have in its place. These two forces find it impossible to merge, because their vibrations are not in resonance with each other. This is a disparity that EFT can correct. It then allows us to attract health, better material circumstances, love, or whatever else we yearn for, with no other real effort required. Things then proceed quite naturally.

BODY AND MIND

The mind and the body form an intimately integrated whole that is indivisible. Our thoughts (beliefs and emotions) dwell throughout our entire body. Because of this, our physical sufferings often have their own stories to tell. A backache can signify that we have had enough of carrying the full responsibility for a household, or a pain in the knee can be a statement that we need to stop for a moment to think about our life. In other words, the body notifies us when the time has come to make significant changes.

Our deepest feelings, with all their repressed needs, often show themselves in the form of physical pain. But their emotional content is of small importance because, from the perspective of EFT, they are always the result of energy blockages. Once these blockages have been removed, the connections may eventually be revealed to us, but becoming aware of them is not required; it is only useful as a matter of curiosity.

THE SUBCONSCIOUS MIND

We all have an ally: the subconscious mind. This is an immensely powerful companion provided to us by nature to help us travel through life in the greatest possible comfort. In the ideal situation, its role consists of applying its phenomenal powers to help us achieve our dreams. Our role is to clearly indicate to it just what those dreams are.

Other than providing this clarity in our requests, there should not be much left for us to do, other than to take advantage of life—our dream life, of course!

However, we are more often ill and starved for love or money than we are satisfied and happy. This suffering is entirely the result of ignorance. Quite often we are not even aware that this collaborator is living inside us, or we are not skilled at putting its expertise to work to our benefit. This is why it heads in one direction, busy with matters it considers important, while we go off in the other direction, concerned with tasks we believe are equally essential. This divergence creates an exhausting conflict, from which we always emerge the loser.

No one can say for sure where the subconscious resides in the human body. But we do know, and have known since the advent of meridian techniques, that the pieces of information it holds are at the very least anchored in our energy system. EFT allows us to go there at a steady pace to alter our suffering at our convenience.

Our subconscious mind has absolute control over everything that happens (or does not happen) in our lives. It is what brings us ideas, tells us how we should conduct ourselves in this or that situation, determines who we meet or don't meet, and opens a door for us over here while shutting another one over there. It is also our subconscious mind that causes us to continually repeat the same mistakes. But this is not because of a malicious intent but solely for our own protection. Our subconscious mind is actually obsessed with protecting us. If it could, it would imprison us and throw away the key, so as not to run the risk of something bad happening to us. And most certainly we are already locked up somewhere. All we need to do to realize it is to write up a list of our problems.

Everything stems from the fact that our subconscious mind follows the directive we give it in our moments of weakness. So if the first experience of speaking in public is too terrifying, for instance, it becomes impossible for us to henceforth speak in public. If our subconscious mind has a lesser opinion of our merits, as a result of various betrayals and other misguided notions about our true skills, we are unlikely, for example, to earn a larger salary.

THE SUBCONSCIOUS AND PROBLEMS

If there is a domain in which everything appears to work against us, it is clearly that of our problems. They arrive, obviously outside of any direct action on our part, and spoil our lives with blatant unfairness. We were so happy before, but that tranquillity is now gone. Armed and ready, we then engage in a fearless battle. We won't go down without a good fight! However, if we are overwhelmed and exhausted by all the battles we have already waged, or if we just don't know what else to do, we remain rooted to one spot, desperately waiting for help. Each time we look outward for solutions, not knowing that our problems—and their solutions—reside within our subconscious mind, which is solely responsible for both.

To get a better grasp of this, let's say that our parents have expressed great animosity toward our artistic talent because it would cause us to abandon the path they had envisioned for us. We decide, nonetheless, to continue on the artistic path we have previously chosen, but all of a sudden, things no longer go as they once did. Doors that were once wide open suddenly slam shut, our creativity withers, and our talents suffer. In short, problems arise, often followed by blistering self-attacks. We obviously lack any talent; this is clearly the proof.

In one sense we are right. We have lost our talents. They are no longer accessible to us because our subconscious mind has shut the door on them to protect one part of the self. This part is the well-behaved child who does not want to disobey his or her parents, whether out of love and respect or out of fear of reprisals. The unpleasant turn of events is therefore not the real problem. It is the childish mind-set that lurks behind it, preventing us from advancing in our adult life as we wish. This is how we end up being robbed of our possibilities in life. Our talents can remain dormant for an entire lifetime beneath the wing of an imperturbable subconscious.

This opposition of the subconscious is so common in people's lives that it has a name in EFT practice. It is called a "psychological reversal," which is treated at the beginning of every session in order to put the subconscious mind in tune with the conscious wishes of the individual. Without this intervention, the tapping sequences may have little to no effect almost half the time.

INTERNAL OPPOSITIONS

These internal oppositions or psychological reversals are the cause for all setbacks. Sensational opportunities are ruined as quickly as possible, exams are failed against all odds, weight that's lost is gained right back, with some people putting on more weight than they started with. These situations can be readily attributed to bad luck or lack of will, although the actual fault always goes back to the data stored in our subconscious mind. If someone seems doomed to remain forever fat or financially challenged, more diets or more money will not change a thing.

All of this takes place unbeknownst to us in the mysterious depths of our energy system. And this is exactly where EFT can work to make the necessary corrections.

EFT AND PROBLEMS

EFT does not address the cause of our problems, which are rooted in the subconscious mind, but concentrates on the energy blockages that correspond to them throughout the energy system. Once these blockages have been dissolved, the true cause of the problem disappears, along with the problem itself.

It is no longer a matter of bravely conquering our fears, or diving to the depths of the grief or shame caused by a situation. It is even possible to circle around a problem from a distance, drawing closer over a course of Tapping sessions as its emotional intensity diminishes, until it disappears completely. A single session is sometimes enough to remove problems that have been receiving conventional therapeutic treatment for months or even years.

EFT AND NEGATIVE EMOTIONS

As Gary Craig has often said, "All negative emotions come from a disruption in our body's energy system." In this conceptualization, negative emotions are not treated as adversaries that must be immediately annihilated. To the contrary, they are allies that are embraced and completely accepted, because they act as a bridge. They are an absolutely essential link to the corresponding energy blockages that need to be removed from our energy system.

All our negative reactions are due to these energy blockages. Often very old, they were ensconced in our energy system over the course of traumatic events, events that may have been too shocking to be processed normally. Following an initial traumatic event, the slightest thing that evokes the memory of it will trigger the blockage associated with it, immediately producing the energetic disruptions that are responsible for our negative feelings.

The energy system can be compared to a television set. As long as the transmission is steady and everything inside it is functioning properly, the sound and images will be clear. But as soon as something goes wrong, static or a fuzzy picture will appear. The television set will display its personal version of a negative emotion.

In the same way, an incident that has disrupted the harmonious flow of energy throughout our energy system produces a kind of buzzing that is responsible for our negative emotions. This famous "zzzzz" is the intermediate stage between a memory and the emotional pain its evocation inflicts, or the one between an event and our negative reactions. Without the energy blockages that produce this zzzzz that is the primary focus of EFT, there are no feelings of terror at the idea of undertaking something challenging, or feelings of anger in response to the actions of others, or feelings of grief from recalling a previously painful memory.

THE RESULTS OF EFT

The emotional intensity of a problem, or the length of time it has been in existence, has no relevance in the practice of EFT. Its cause always lies in the energy blockages that disrupt the harmonious functioning of the bioenergy system. Extremely old problems are no more deeply rooted in this system than new ones. The complexity comes from the number of aspects a problem may have, each of which represents one energy blockage. Rounds of tapping on every possible angle are then necessary to solve the problem.

EFT provides extremely quick results in the treatment of phobias and numerous pains connected to the memories of tragic events. Feelings of horror, terror, guilt, or heart-rending separation are dissolved and replaced by a sense of deep tranquillity.

On the other hand, problems with tentacles that extend into many aspects of our lives, such as a chronic lack of money or a disastrous relationship, take more time to resolve. Persistent use of EFT is called for to remove all the mental boundaries and restrictive beliefs that have led to these kinds of situations. There may also be important decisions to make and significant turning points that should not be rushed into. In these cases results may take longer to manifest. But they will manifest, that is certain. The Peace Procedure offers a solid guarantee of this (see page 42). Persistence truly pays off in the practice of EFT. It is a simple technique that nevertheless requires the correct approach for best results, so for thornier challenges, it may be advisable to work initially with a therapist who can help you in that regard.

In the case of a recurring problem, the problem may keep cropping up because its roots have not been treated, so another aspect of it keeps appearing. Several tapping sequences will be required to eliminate a new aspect of the problem. So, for example, you have lost your fear of spiders after having been successfully treated earlier, but your fear suddenly reappears when one of these creatures rushes toward you. This indicates that an aspect of the phobia has not yet been treated, but one or two rounds of tapping should be enough to eliminate it completely.

EFT offers excellent results for physical problems. It is a choice addition to any kind of treatment because of its ability to regulate the flow of energy through the body. It is an undeniable fact that emotional suffering contributes to physical suffering. Because of this, the elimination of one often removes the other as well.

2
The EFT Protocol

A complete EFT sequence can be performed in less than a minute. The shorter version can take a mere twenty seconds. Both the shorter and longer versions are performed in the same way—in five successive stages. What distinguishes them is the number of points to be stimulated. It is perfectly fine to use the shorter version, but it is a good idea to also know the complete version, which can be quite helpful if you do not achieve the progress you were hoping for with the shorter version.

SUMMARY OF THE FIVE STEPS
TO AN EFT SEQUENCE

1. Concentration on the problem
2. Evaluation of the intensity of the pain
3. The setup that momentarily causes inner barriers to fall
4. The tapping sequence accompanied by the reminder phrase that keeps the problem in the forefront of your mind
5. Reevaluation of the intensity of the pain at the end of

the sequence to determine how much progress has been made

CONCENTRATION

Focusing attention on a negative emotion that is caused by an energy blockage rooted in the energy system helps maintain the activity of the turbulence until the blockage can be dissolved. Without setting up this specific target, the tapping will fire into the void and have no effect.

EVALUATION

The purpose of EFT is to completely eliminate a painful emotion or source of physical suffering. The evaluation is used to estimate the intensity of the pain before each round of tapping so that whatever progress is made can be assessed at the end. In EFT terminology, this evaluation step is called identifying the "subjective units of distress," or SUD.

The evaluation is made using a scale of 0 to 10, the number 10 representing an intense emotional or physical pain, and 0 representing its complete disappearance. It is important to rate the level of suffering as it is experienced at the actual moment of beginning the tapping round, and not to base it on past feelings or hope for relief at a later time. The first number that comes to mind is generally the most accurate. Use this figure to evaluate your progress, even if you are not sure it is correct. In a less precise way you can also assess the intensity of a pain by defining it as weak, moderate, or strong.

THE SETUP

The setup is a crucial stage that is used to eliminate the psychological reversal mentioned earlier. This step prepares the energy system. It corrects reversals of polarity that are created when the subconscious mind opposes our desire to change, pushing the energy to circulate in the wrong direction. It's similar to what happens when AA batteries are installed upside down; they cannot make the connection. Polarity reversal is not connected to our energy blockages, but as it is often present, its remedy is always included in the standard EFT sequence.

You create the setup by saying a phrase that *specifically* expresses the emotion or physical pain you hope to remove, while simultaneously stimulating a point that corrects the energetic polarity. The phrase stipulates that you accept yourself entirely despite any flaws, problems, and deficiencies you perceive in your life. This affirmation brings a halt to inner struggle for a moment, which is just enough time to perform a liberating round of tapping with no interference from the subconscious mind. For example, for a pain you could say, "I accept myself completely, even though my shoulder hurts."

If you find this phrase of accepting yourself and your

problems difficult to believe, don't worry; you are not the only one. In this case you can regard this step like a game, without worrying about the veracity of the statement. The important thing is the treatment that will take place in your energy system as you say these words. Massage of the Sore Spot or vigorous tapping on the Karate Chop point will reverse the energetic polarity and take care of your resistance even when you would normally find it hard to say that you accepted yourself completely in a particular situation.

The phrase is always constructed the same way; the only thing that changes is the segment concerning the problem. Here are some other examples: "I accept myself completely, even though I have a fear of speaking in public." "I accept myself completely, even though I failed my exam." "I accept myself completely, even though I am feeling this anger," and so forth.

You should repeat the phrase three times in a row, preferably aloud, with as much emphasis as possible, while circularly massaging (in a clockwise direction) the Sore Spot or vigorously tapping the Karate Chop point (see the illustrations on pages 24 and 25) and at the same time focusing your attention on the physical pain or emotion expressed in your statement.

To find the Sore Spot, place your hand at the base of your throat at the spot where a tie would be knotted. Go down about three inches, then look for this point another three inches to the left (or to the right, if you prefer). You will find it somewhere in this area. Some people may feel a fairly sharp pain when pressing on it, while others may hardly feel it. It depends on the congestion of the lymphatic system because this point has no connection to the meridian network.

The Karate Chop point can be found on the cutting edge of the hand between the base of the little finger and the start of the wrist, the place that is used in martial arts practice for breaking an object with a sharp blow. This point should be struck vigorously with the flat part of the fingers on your other hand.

It is preferable to stimulate the Sore Spot, but the Karate Chop point will restore energetic polarity very effectively as well. Of course, you will not use the Sore Spot if, for the slightest reason, you are not able to apply any pressure on this part of your body. In this case, use the Karate Chop point.

TAPPING: THE REMINDER PHRASE ROUND

Immediately following the setup that momentarily lowers your internal resistance, you must quickly begin the round of tapping, the liberating step of EFT.

One round is performed by lightly tapping, with the tips of the index and middle fingers, the series of points described later, while repeating a short reminder phrase of the problem, one time only, at each point. This reminder keeps the subconscious mind aware of the particular blockage you are seeking to eliminate. In other words, it holds the target securely in the right place.

This reminder consists of the segment of the setup phrase connected to the problem. For example, for a phrase such as "I accept myself completely, even though I have this fear of speaking in public," the reminder phrase in the statement is "this fear of speaking in public." The reminder phrase is spoken at each point of the sequence, while your attention remains fully focused on the accompanying emotion.

The Points of the Tapping Round

The tapping round is a descending sequence that travels down from the face to the hands. You can use either hand to tap the points, or even change hands midway, and you can stimulate the points on the side of the body that is most convenient. You can even change sides at any time during the sequence if you desire. You must give between seven and ten light taps to each point, depending on the length of the reminder phrase (but no fewer than five). But you should not count the number of taps during the sequence, as counting will impede the concentration you need to focus on your problem.

THE COMPLETE THREE-PART TAPPING ROUND

The complete version of a round of tapping is put together much like a sandwich: one round of tapping, the Gamut point procedure, and then another round of tapping.

Part 1: Initial Tapping Points of the Round

1. **Eyebrow:** located at the beginning of the eyebrow at the side of the nose.

2. **Side of the eye:** located on the eye socket bone at the end of the eyebrow.

3. **Under the eye:** located on the eye socket bone directly vertical to the pupil when you are looking straight ahead.

4. **Under the nose:** located at the center of the space between the nose and the upper lip.

5. **Hollow of the chin:** located between the lower lip and the bump of the chin.

6. **Collarbone:** located to the right or left of the central "V" that connects the two collarbones, right beneath the protuberance of the bone. This point is struck by the tips of the five fingers and more sharply than the other points.

7. **Underarm:** located on the side of the chest about four inches beneath the armpit, right where a bra would encircle the body. This point can be tapped with the tips of all five fingers.

8. **Under the breast:** located below the breast in line with the nipple of both men and women.

9. **Thumb:** located at the edge of the thumbnail on the outer side of your hand.

10. **Index finger:** located at the base of the nail on the side facing the thumb.

11. **Middle finger:** located at the base of the nail on the side facing the thumb.

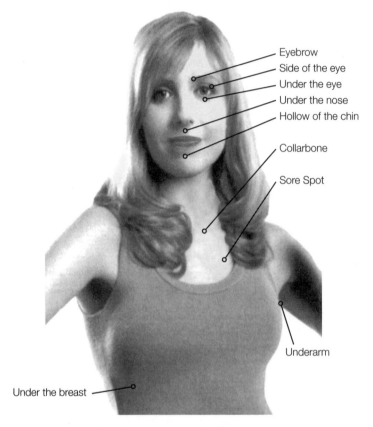

Eyebrow
Side of the eye
Under the eye
Under the nose
Hollow of the chin

Collarbone

Sore Spot

Underarm

Under the breast

Tapping points on the face and chest

12. **Little finger:** located at the base of the nail on the side facing the thumb.

13. **Karate Chop point:** located on the outside edge of the hand between the base of the little finger and the wrist, the place that is used in martial arts practice when breaking an object with one sharp strike of the hand. Strike this point vigorously with the flats of the fingers of the other hand.

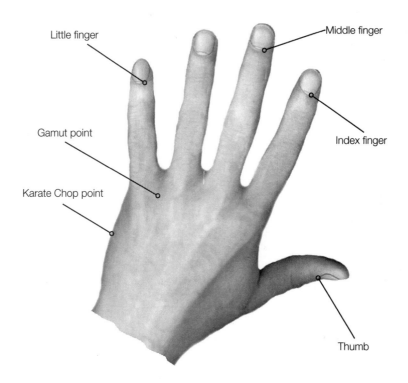

Tapping points on the hand

The preceding section is the first part of a complete round of Tapping, similar to the first slice of bread for a sandwich.

Part 2: The Gamut Point Procedure

We shall now look at the protocol of the Gamut point, which is layered in the center of the tapping round. This is a procedure that balances the two hemispheres of the brain, allowing the energy system to dissolve a blockage more easily in the case of resistance.

It is first necessary to find the Gamut point. It is located on the top of the hand, in the "V" that is formed by drawing a triangle down from the base of the ring finger and little finger. This zone should be struck with the flat parts of the fingers of the other hand while you keep your mind fixed on your problem and go through the entire nine-step sequence of the Gamut point. This sequence is performed as follows:

1. Close your eyes.
2. Open your eyes.
3. Look down to the right while keeping your head steady.
4. Look down to the left while keeping your head steady.
5. Roll your eyes in a complete circle without moving your head.
6. Roll your eyes in a complete circle again, in the opposite direction.
7. Hum some bars of a familiar song for three seconds.
8. Quickly count from one to five.
9. Hum the same song again for three seconds.

Part 3: Final Tapping Points of the Round

Once the middle of the sequence has been achieved with the completion of the Gamut point procedure, repeat the first part of the round again, stimulating the same points from 1 to 13.

1. **Eyebrow:** located at the beginning of the eyebrow at the side of the nose.

2. **Side of the eye:** located on the eye socket bone at the end of the eyebrow.

3. **Under the eye:** located on the eye socket bone directly vertical to the pupil when you are looking straight ahead.

4. **Under the nose:** located at the center of the space between the nose and the upper lip.

5. **Hollow of the chin:** located between the lower lip and the bump of the chin.

6. **Collarbone:** located to the right or left of the central "V" that connects the two collarbones, right beneath the protuberance of the bone. This point is struck by the tips of the five fingers and more sharply than the other points.

7. **Underarm:** located on the side of the chest about four inches beneath the armpit, right where a bra would encircle the body. This point can be tapped with the tips of all five fingers.

8. **Under the breast:** located below the breast in line with the nipple of both men and women.

9. **Thumb:** located at the edge of the thumbnail on the outer side of your hand.

10. **Index finger:** located at the base of the nail on the side facing the thumb.

11. **Middle finger:** located at the base of the nail on the side facing the thumb.

12. **Little finger:** located at the base of the nail on the side facing the thumb.

13. **Karate Chop point:** located on the outside edge of the hand between the base of the little finger and the

wrist, the place that is used in martial arts practice when breaking an object with one sharp strike of the hand. Strike this point vigorously with the flats of the fingers of the other hand.

The Abbreviated EFT Round of Tapping

The shortened round includes only the points of the face down to the point on the torso beneath the breast, or numbers 1 through 8. All the others points of the longer version are omitted, although you can always choose to incorporate them in the event that progress comes to a halt.

As all the meridians are interdependent, stimulating one necessarily engages the others, and those on the fingers are also inevitably stimulated as they are used as the instruments for tapping. For the short sequence of EFT, follow the normal steps of the setup and evaluation, but tap only the first eight points:

1. **Eyebrow:** located at the beginning of the eyebrow at the side of the nose.
2. **Side of the eye:** located on the eye socket bone at the end of the eyebrow.
3. **Under the eye:** located on the eye socket bone directly vertical to the pupil when you are looking straight ahead.
4. **Under the nose:** located at the center of the space between the nose and the upper lip.
5. **Hollow of the chin:** located between the lower lip and the bump of the chin.

6. **Collarbone:** located to the right or left of the central "V" that connects the two collarbones, right beneath the protuberance of the bone. This point is struck by the tips of the five fingers and more sharply than the other points.

7. **Underarm:** located on the side of the chest about four inches beneath the armpit, right where a bra would encircle the body. This point can be tapped with the tips of all five fingers.

8. **Under the breast:** located below the breast in line with the nipple of both men and women.

REEVALUATION

This step is used to evaluate the progress made during the round of tapping that has just been completed. If your starting level of distress was a 7, did you reach a serene 0 when you ended the round? A 3 or a 5? Did you remain stuck in place with an inflexible 7? Perhaps you even moved up in the scale to an 8 or 10? Failure to achieve the relief you had anticipated can usually be attributed to one or more of the the following reasons:

- Your attention was scattered during the Tapping round, so the arrow (EFT) missed its target (the problem).
- You did not describe your problem with enough precision during the setup stage, or you did not use the right words (or the most raw words), or you failed to

employ the necessary emphasis when you said it aloud.

- Another aspect of the problem appeared (the aspects are explained in greater detail later).
- Your subconscious mind realized that a liberating event was occurring and reactivated your defenses before the tapping round had time to take effect.

THE FOLLOWING ROUNDS

You may wish to perform more rounds to obtain the desired relief. The setup differs in the following rounds because the progress made in the previous sequence is taken into account. Even if the reevaluation figure is higher or remains identical to the initial figure, the setup phrase should be modified to focus on the aspects of the problem that remain to be treated. The repetition of the modified setup phase allows us to get a sense of the progress that has already been made or, if we have not seen progress, it serves to win the agreement of our subconscious mind by reassuring it of our desire for change.

Let's say you began the first round with a setup phrase such as this: "I accept myself completely, even though I am feeling immense anger." You might construct the setup statement for the following round by using the phrase "I accept myself completely, even though I am still feeling immense anger," and then you could use "even though I still feel what is left of the anger" for each of the following rounds until you have established a state of internal calm. EFT does not alter the reality of things; it simply dissolves the emotional charge (energy blockage) connected to an event.

HOW AN EFT SESSION UNFOLDS

Let's begin by choosing an event—one that is short and precise—that still evokes negative feelings every time you think of it. It might be an odious remark, a slap you received as a child, an incident that caused you great fear, or any other painful memory. You can also decide to treat a physical pain. The pathwork is identical for all kinds of problems.

Write down the gist of your problem in a short phrase as if it were the title of a movie—for example, *The Pain in My Left Shoulder, Stuck in the Elevator,* or *Mary's Criticism.*

Now evaluate the level of your suffering from this problem on a scale going from 0 to 10, with 10 being indicative of the ultimate pain and 0 its utter disappearance. Write down your number next to the title of your problem.

We now come to the step of the setup that removes the opposition of your subconscious in the event that your subconscious would prefer to have you hang on to your problem. This state, as mentioned earlier, is called a psychological reversal, and if it has not been dealt with at the beginning of the sequence, it often prevents the rounds from having their desired effect.

Perform this corrective step by saying the phrase of your complete acceptance of yourself and your problem *three times in a row,* while stimulating the Sore Spot or the

Karate Chop point. Stimulate whichever point you prefer, as they are interchangeable.

This setup stage is always constructed in the same way. It opens with your expression of self-acceptance despite your problem, which you should describe as precisely as possible: "I accept myself completely, even though . . . (here you *specifically* describe your problem)." For example, you might say, "I accept myself completely, even though I am feeling immense anger," or "I accept myself completely, even though my father spanked me on my seventh birthday."

Your subconscious mind is now ready to help you resolve your problem. But you must get started with the tapping round right away before it throws up the usual barriers again.

Here, you can stimulate all the points of the full EFT round (see pages 22–28) or you can use the shortcut version (pages 28–29). Begin with the short version, but then immediately perform the complete version if your pain is not reduced.

The tapping rounds are performed as you repeat (only once) a short reminder phrase at each stimulation point. For the examples cited above, it would be "immense anger" or "my father spanked me," while you concentrate as strongly as possible on the emotions you are feeling.

A reevaluation is necessary next to determine how much progress was made during the round you just completed. If you have not achieved the relief you desire, continue performing the rounds.

During the next rounds, the setup statement will be different because you will be taking into account the progress that was made during the preceding round, even if it is not truly perceptible. Let's take as our example the problem of feeling immense anger. The next setup will take place by saying: "I accept myself completely, even though I am still feeling immense anger."

For your specific problem, you can say: "I accept myself completely, even though I am still feeling . . . (example: this pain in my left knee)," or "I accept myself completely, even though I am still at an 8 in . . . (example: my deep grief at the death of my animal companion)."

This will be the new setup phrase that you will repeat three times in succession (with as much emphasis as possible) while massaging the Sore Spot or striking the Karate Chop point. The reminder phrase of the following round will stipulate the part of the problem that remains to be treated—for example, "what remains of the pain in my left knee," or "this 8 that remains of my grief for my animal companion."

It is sometimes necessary to go through several rounds before all the emotional suffering has dissipated. This repetition often meants that different aspects of the problem need to be treated individually.

3
Working with EFT

The biggest challenge in EFT is figuring out how many rounds of tapping should be administered.

THE ASPECTS

Gary Craig, the creator of EFT, compares a problem to a table that has many legs, each of which represents a different aspect of the problem. In order to remove the fundamental cause of the problem, each leg needs to be cut down in succession in order for the top of the table—which represents the problem—to collapse. This task can seem disheartening at first glance, but it is considerably facilitated by the realization that when a number of these legs that hold up the tabletop get knocked down, the remainder (there can be thousands) will fall on their own accord with no additional effort needed.

This is called the "generalization effect" in the practice of EFT. One round eliminates one aspect (one leg of the table), then another aspect comes forth and is eliminated in turn, until the moment when the table (the problem), with all its remaining legs, suddenly falls apart. A solution to the problem then clearly appears, or a profound sense of peace arises to replace the emotional pain.

For the tabletop to exist, a powerful event must have left a deep imprint in the energy system, perhaps quite long ago. From the initial moment forward, the tabletop becomes increasingly sturdy as additional legs are incorporated to consolidate its footing. These legs are formed every time flagrant proof of the problem is displayed again. For example, for abandonment issues, every time an event causes us to feel that we have been excluded or rejected, we form a new table leg.

EFT's ability to intervene in specific events is part of its winning formula, because it can be done at any time, in any situation, without someone else's help. Starting the process for a lack of self-confidence or deep-seated loneliness can provide momentary relief but will not remove the deep cause of the problem. To truly eliminate it, the specific aspects of the situation must be treated. In other words, one or more of the tapping sequences should be performed during evocation of an event that provides evidence of the problem as a whole.

For example, a lack of self-confidence could manifest on a day when you were petrified by shyness in the presence of someone you deemed important. Intolerable loneliness may stem from a sad Christmas Eve spent without friends or family a long time ago. All these painful feelings, felt at the evocation of these specific events, should then be the subject of separately performed rounds.

To return to the example of deep grief connected to the death of an animal companion, let's say that the grief has not diminished over the course of the first three rounds. There would be no sense in continuing to work in an overly general way. Various aspects (energy blockages) are contributing to the grief and need to be eliminated one by one. In this case they might be anger at the veterinarian for poor treatment, guilt for not having had the knowledge or perhaps the funds to give your pet better treatment, the memory of your companion's gentle nature or magnificent gaze, and so on and so forth. Tapping rounds would address each of these until it is possible to say, in all tranquillity, "My beloved companion is gone and I will never see him (or her) again, but all is well."

Don't make the error of practicing EFT on generalities. Without wanting to, you may considerably delay your emotional healing and risk becoming weary of the procedure in very short order. This would be too bad, because EFT otherwise is rapid and effective. If you are not achieving the results you desire, you may also want to consider working with a professional EFT practitioner.

WORKING ALONE WITH EFT

The best way of working alone with EFT is with a pencil and a piece of paper. The subsequent session will unfold in a way that makes it easier to get to the heart of the problem. You will not go astray while following your path. Each step fits into the next to govern painful beliefs as they make their appearance. These beliefs are still connected to different energy blockages, which will melt away over the course of the Tapping rounds.

The process begins by identifying the problem, such as, for example, a conflict with someone, a habit of always being late, or a fear of public speaking in the near future. The beginning of the session incorporates the elements of the problem in the setup and an evaluation of the pain, followed by the round accompanied with a reminder. Let's say here, "I accept myself completely even though I am fearful about making this speech," with the reminder "fearful of making this speech."

As other beliefs and memories arise, they can be written down on paper, each supplying the reason for a round or two of Tapping. The session ends with a new statement of the problem, such as "I am afraid of making this speech," at which point the participant generally notices that the statement is no longer true; the fear has dissipated and has been replaced by pleasant feelings such as self-confidence. The real test will obviously take place during the speech, which has every chance of being made with the greatest ease.

Following treatment of the problem, you will often see that it no longer has any hold on you, and you may even wonder how it could have upset you as much as it formerly did. This is one of the customary effects of EFT.

We can even forget the essence of the problem that was just treated.

HOW TO CHOOSE GOOD EFT SETUP PHRASES

The setup phrases always incorporate the specific substance of the problem, which is very personal for each individual. For this reason it is not feasible to have a manual that lists every problem and appropriate setup phrases. Such a list could address only general issues, whereas specificity is essential for EFT to be effective.

Let's take as an example a conflict issue we are having with a colleague at work named Marcel. The first setup phrase will begin with acceptance of the problem: "I accept myself completely, even though I have this conflict with Marcel" (for which the reminder phrase would be "this conflict with Marcel"). Then we will move on to the actual emotions we are feeling by using whatever words we feel necessary, including the most crude, during the following setups: "I accept myself completely, even though I hate this moron Marcel," or "I accept myself completely, even though I really want to get him fired," and so on, while performing as many rounds as necessary to eliminate the hatred or the desire for revenge that accompanies the phrases cited above. The profound elements that caused the conflict will also dissolve, thus restoring a peaceful work environment.

With EFT we never beat around the bush. We look

for the most negative feelings in order to achieve the most thorough eradication of them all. In this way we reach a point by the end of the session where we can see things in a way that is serene and impartial.

EFT AND THE MEMORY OF TRAGIC EVENTS

When events prove impossible to forget, it is because conclusions drawn from the events have remained anchored in our energy system, producing the disruptions responsible for our torment. Feelings of fear, hatred, anger, injustice, powerlessness, guilt, or despair, as well as physical pain, insomnia, and nightmares, can all be part and parcel of an inner upheaval that may last a lifetime if left untreated.

EFT leads to a sense of tranquillity over the course of a series of rounds, the number of which will depend on the quantity of aspects to be treated with respect to the entire episode. For witnesses to a fast-moving event, such as the attack on the World Trade Center, these aspects will be tied to various outstanding facts of the catastrophe. However, for a war veteran, for example, these aspects might be associated with a large number of tragic stories over a sustained period of time.

Treatment begins with the first memory that comes to mind, followed by another, and then another, in a series of rounds that will eventually eliminate the emotional charge. The narration technique that will be described in greater depth on page 66 is the most effective means of using EFT for getting rid of the suffering attached to memories.

EFT AND PHOBIAS

All phobic responses are caused by an energetic disruption that can be eliminated quite easily by EFT. To eliminate a phobia, it is important to treat all its aspects. For example, in regard to a fear of flying, there are fears of taking off, landing, turbulence, and having no control over the engine, as well as the fear that the plane will fall from the sky, of being trapped with no way out, and so on, as a sample of all the painful beliefs that can be associated with the idea of traveling by airplane, including bad memories.

In a panic situation, several rounds of Tapping should suffice to rapidly restore a sense of calm. Knowing that you have this tool available at any time provides a sense of courage that is otherwise not available.

EFT AND ADDICTIVE BEHAVIORS

The true reason for these needy behaviors has to do with deep anxiety. This is a pain that an individual may temporarily mask with a substance of choice, carrying out a tenuous treatment that could develop into dependency.

EFT does not address this dependency, but it does address its profound cause—an anxiety, and therefore a negative emotion—which is simply an energy blockage. But while the treatment is simple, the opposition put up by the subconscious mind can complicate matters significantly.

The psychological reversal we discussed earlier almost always accompanies dependencies. This will require frequent treatment during the first few days after the individual has quit taking the addictive substance. The treatment for each craving takes place during the setup stage of the EFT sequence, followed by rounds of Tapping for as long as all the energy blockages responsible for the feeling of anxiety persist.

Without this subconscious opposition, correcting the reversal of the energy polarity continuously at the beginning of the treatment with one or two rounds of EFT could be enough to cause an addictive need to vanish forever.

Given the fact that EFT heals the anxiety responsible for the dependency, there is no risk of developing a new dependency to replace the one that has been eliminated, nor of taking on the pounds of additional weight that are a well-known consequence of quitting smoking and various substances.

EFT AND PHYSICAL PAIN

Pain management is probably one of the most requested needs of people seeking relief, and EFT responds to this demand in an amazing way. Without going into great detail from the case studies that are available on the official EFT website (www.emofree.com), suffice it to say that there are

countless people who have received help from EFT for easier breathing, release of a stiff neck or sore back, an allergy,
or a migraine.

The treatment uses the standard EFT sequence. The
intensity of the pain is evaluated, followed by a setup such
as "I accept myself completely, even though I have this stiff
neck," with the reminder phrase "this stiff neck" during
the Tapping round.

As is customary, subsequent sequences take into
account the remnant of the pain to be treated, with one
particular feature that needs to be stressed. At this point
the pain may move around the body. This is so common in
EFT practice that it has given rise to the expression "chas-
ing the pain." It is a kind of traveling pain that needs to be
pursued by multiple rounds until all the energy blockages
responsible for it have been removed.

Physical pains can also have a message to give us. All
you need to do is to ask them the question. Then perform
Tapping rounds on the ideas that cross through your mind,
including even those you may find completely absurd.

The EFT Peace Procedure

The Peace Procedure consists of making a list of all
the difficult incidents that have occurred in your life.
This period should span the time from earliest childhood to five years ago, as your emotional experience of the most recent five years is always a repeat

of your emotional experience of older events. Next EFT is applied to each of them until their memory no longer inspires any painful feeling. Fear, sorrow, and anger have all been replaced by a deep sense of tranquillity.

It is imperative to write down at least one hundred events, and even more if possible. Take your time. You can always begin treating the first memories without waiting to complete your list, but don't be surprised if you have trouble getting started. The subconscious mind is hardly eager for change. While it is wonderfully well adapted to our life circumstances, it can oppose our desire for healing and transformation if it decides that there are too many risks involved.

If you do not manage to complete this list, despite your best intentions, do several rounds of Tapping on this obvious internal opposition. Use setup phrases such as "I accept myself completely, even though I have not managed to make my list yet," or "I accept myself completely, even though I never have the desire (or time) to practice EFT."

Every event notation should be short and focused. A situation that lasted several hours, or even several days, is comprised of different episodes that are to be treated separately. They are separate aspects of the same problem.

Write down the facts quite precisely. Do not say,

"My father is abusive," but go into the details of specific events, such as "My father gave me a violent spanking in the kitchen," or "he took my bicycle away from me," or "he belittled me in front of my friends."

Treat one event at a time until the entire emotional charge it carries has evaporated. In the case where it is difficult to reduce, do several rounds of Tapping on all the angles of the situation. Work on a specific event takes only several moments, so working at this pace, within three months you can erase the painful mark left by one hundred difficult events. You can already imagine the benefits. The ideal would be to devote fifteen minutes to the procedure every day, and more if you can.

4

A Collection of
Painful Statements

The goal of EFT is to heal all your inner wounds, for the less grief, fear, and anger you carry buried within you, the better you will feel. For this reason we have assembled a collection of painful statements with the intention of helping you to rediscover your bad memories, so that you can remove the imprint that remains stamped in your energy system.

The negative sentences offered in this collection are generalities. They are typical vague assertions that EFT can rarely sweep away in one swoop. To repeat our earlier metaphor of a table, a bad memory or traumatic event (represented in these statements) forms the tabletop, which is supported by numerous legs, each of which represents a specific event that confirms the statement in question.

Out of these following general statements, choose the ones that best apply to your personal suffering. Write them down with all the supporting evidence, as if you were trying to convince someone. Then perform Tapping rounds on each event until the emotional charge has vanished completely.

PAINFUL STATEMENTS

These are general statements, with examples. Each of us has had unique life experiences, so feel free to elaborate or vary from the words listed, so that the statement feels true for you. If you've ever had someone massage you, you know there is often a sensitive spot, sometimes called a "trigger point," that seems to be the epicenter of some discomfort. Words, too, can have a trigger point, so you may want to play with these statements until you discover one that hits on that kind of a sensitive spot for you.

I feel abandoned (rejected, excluded, repressed, neglected).

I have been betrayed (unjustly accused, denounced, slandered, dishonored, attacked).

I was mistreated as a child (tormented, humiliated, bullied).

I was denied love (affection, care, tenderness).

Happiness is not in the cards for me (I gave up a long time ago, I will never get out of this, I can't win).

I have lost everything that was dear to me (I am inconsolable, beaten down, depressed).

I am completely absorbed by my problems (I find satisfaction in recounting my misfortunes, and sharing them with others, and nobody suffers the way I do).

I always leave decisions up to others (I avoid making decisions, I never impose my wishes on anyone).

I must do everything on my own (no one is there to protect me or support me, nobody cares about me).

I do not know how to ask for help (I am unable to express my needs or even admit that I have them).

I did not educate my children properly (I am a bad mother, my children don't share their lives with me, I have no connection with my children).

I carry a heavy secret (I have things to be ashamed for, I have contributed to my own downfall, I'm guilty).

I do not trust anyone (I do not confide in anyone, I never show weakness, I would never accept help).

People are despicable (cruel, dishonest, violent, selfish, greedy).

No one has ever helped me find the right path (I don't have the education necessary to succeed, nobody taught me how to do things right).

I am used to suffering (I will never get better, this problem can't be solved).

I will never get what I want (I'll never have enough money, I'll always be single, I'm not meant to be happy).

Nothing good ever happens to me (everything always turns sour, everything always takes a turn for the worse, I'm unlucky).

I have gotten rid of all my desire for pleasure (love, money, affection).

I am not accepted by others (I'm different, shocking, eccentric, weird).

I am insignificant (invisible, my opinion is of no value, nobody cares what I think or do).

I have every flaw imaginable (for example, I'm selfish, mean, unlovable, obnoxious, and so on) and I have proof of it (list the proof).

I am hated by _____ (the individual's name).

I detest _____ (the individual's name).

I am too stupid (too ugly, old, big, small, fat, thin, weird, nerdy, awkward).

I cannot break my promise (I made a pact, my life is not my own, I made my bed and I have to lie in it).

I will never get free of this debt (of these obligations, this promise).

I am scared of losing (of lacking something, failing, looking bad).

I am scared of solitude (of loneliness, separation, confrontations, being watched).

I'm scared of getting fat (of losing my hair, falling ill, getting old, being broke).

I'm scared of speaking in public (of strangers, being far from home, trying new things).

I'm scared of the dark (of crowds, cramped spaces, being trampled, heights, flying).

I'm scared of losing control (of my money, my children, my spouse, my house).

I'm scared of rats (snakes, spiders, birds, dogs, cats).

STATING THE POSITIVE BY
TAPPING ON THE OCCIPITAL BULGE

A successful EFT session always ends in a vast sensation of inner peace and newfound freedom. This is the perfect time to give your subconscious mind new directives using what is called "positive assertion" by tapping on the occipital bulge. This procedure does not form part of the standard EFT technique, the objective of which is erasure of the negative. It is an add-on that makes it possible to end a session in beauty, while also putting our inner partner on notice regarding the tasks it will henceforth have to do for us.

The occipital bulge is a point on the back of the head where the meridians meet. It is located at the base of the skull, an inch or so above the neck. This bump is easier to find when you lean your head forward.

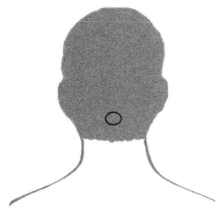

The occipital bulge

Stating the positive is implemented by distinctly saying what you desire while tapping this bump without stopping. Here are a few examples of possible statements:

I feel financially secure now.

Money now comes to me from all directions very easily.

I now clearly see the path to take to achieve success.

I will now pass my exams with honors.

I am now very much at ease when speaking publicly.

Love has entered my life now and is here to stay.

Things will always turn out in my favor now.

Now I will own the car of my dreams.

My career is now blossoming fabulously well.

I am forging ahead with all the support I need now.

I am experiencing a wonderful comeback now.

5

The Body's Meridians and Their Emotional Function

The following quick introduction is offered merely to satisfy your curiosity, because other than complete familiarity with the points used in the tapping sequence, no knowledge of the meridians is required to get effective assistance from EFT.

The meridian lines form a network of channels that carry energy throughout the body. There are fourteen of these meridians in all. Twelve of these meridian channels travel through the various organs from which they take their names and occur as symmetrical yin/yang pairs on both sides of the body. The other two are unilateral and do not follow the "tidal" clock that regulates the paired meridians. The points on the surface of the meridians serve as portals through which the surrounding energy can enter the body and leave again in a continuous coming-and-going movement.

The meridians form a closely connected whole. Each

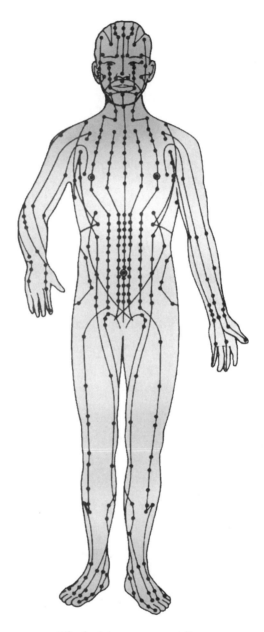

The body's energy meridians

meridian line is, in fact, the particular segment of a single same "river of energy" (with numerous tributaries) that deeply enters the body and resurfaces, in the process changing the yin/yang polarity. The tapping points of EFT are located at these spots where the polarity is reversed, and tapping on them confers a complete treatment of all the meridians. Our physical and emotional health depends upon good movement of energy in this transport system. An energy flow that is too fast or slow, that has been interrupted somewhere, or that is circulating in the wrong direction is the source of all our discomforts.

This concept is summarized in the classic tenet of EFT: all negative emotions are due to a disruption in the body's energy system. These emotions can have an impact on our physical health, as there is no separation between mind and body. With EFT, a physical pain can be reduced by treating an emotional affliction, and vice versa, which is why we focus closely on physical sensations during tapping sequences.

It also explains a very curious phenomenon that often occurs during a sequence, in which the pains begin to travel across the body. These pains are then "chased down" with additional rounds of EFT, to provide the purest possible relief for emotional suffering.

It takes energy twenty-four hours to make a complete circuit of the body. Each section is traversed in two hours, the period of time in which the energy of each organ meridian is most active. Energy is primarily yin in nature when it travels through the yin organs—the heart, spleen-pancreas, lungs, kidneys, and liver. With the exception of the lungs, the yin organs are distinguished primarily by not having empty cavities and their function is to produce, transform, and store fundamental substances (qi, blood, and other body fluids).

The energy is considered primarily yang when it crosses through the visceral organs—organs with empty cavities—including the upper and lower intestines, stomach, urinary bladder, and gallbladder.

Each meridian is named according to the area it travels through, and it is saturated with the energetic personality of the element (from the Chinese five-element cycle) with which it is associated. In the five-element cycle, five elemental phases of energy flow from the interaction of yin and yang. These elements—wood, fire, earth, metal, and water—symbolically express the five tendencies of energy in motion. Wood represents energy that is beginning or developing. Fire represents energy that is expanding. Earth represents energy that is stabilizing. Metal represents energy that is contracting, and water represents energy that is gathering and sinking. Each pair of organ meridians is governed by one of the five elements as follows:

Wood governs the liver and gallbladder.
Fire governs the heart and small intestine (as well as the pair formed by the yin Pericardium, or Heart

Protector, meridian and the yang Triple Warmer meridian).

Earth governs the spleen-pancreas and stomach.

Metal governs the lungs and large intestine.

Water governs the kidneys and urinary bladder.

The timetable (or tidal clock) of meridian activity is as follows:

1:00 a.m. to 3:00 a.m.: Yin—Wood—Liver

3:00 a.m. to 5:00 a.m.: Yin—Metal—Lungs

5:00 a.m. to 7:00 a.m.: Yang—Metal—Large Intestine

7:00 a.m. to 9:00 a.m.: Yang—Earth—Stomach

9:00 a.m. to 11:00 a.m.: Yin—Earth—Spleen-Pancreas

11:00 a.m. to 1:00 p.m.: Yin—Fire—Heart

1:00 p.m. to 3:00 p.m.: Yang—Fire—Small Intestine

3:00 p.m. to 5:00 p.m.: Yang—Water—Urinary Bladder

5:00 p.m. to 7:00 p.m.: Yin—Water—Kidneys

7:00 p.m. to 9:00 p.m.: Yin—Fire—Pericardium (circulation/sex)

9:00 p.m. to 11:00 p.m.: Yang—Fire—Triple Warmer (thyroid)

11:00 p.m. to 1:00 a.m.: Yang—Wood—Gall Bladder

The Functional Channel (or Conception Vessel), which is yin in nature and runs up the front of the body, combines with the Governor Channel (or Governing Vessel), which is yang in nature and runs up the back of the body, to form a separate pair, and they are unilateral. The first controls all of the yin meridians, and the second all of the yang meridians.

EMOTIONAL FUNCTIONS OF THE MERIDIANS ACCORDING TO THE EFT TAPPING POINTS

The Sore Spot

This point, where the EFT sequences begin (unless the individual has a preference for the Karate Chop point), is not located on the meridian network, although its stimulation helps rebalance these lines by retargeting their yin/yang polarity. This point can be found along the lymphatic system and its sensitivity is indicative of a swelling that regular stimulation will generally cause to disappear.

Emotional aim: This point is useful for the freeing of a psychological reversal, or a pact made with the subconscious in favor of protection for a certain period, but which now poses severe restrictions.

The Karate Chop Point

Meridian: Small Intestine (paired with the Heart meridian)

Element: Fire

Emotional aim: The other choice spot (along with the Sore Spot) for emancipation from psychological reversals. Stimulating this point calms feelings of apprehension, anxiety, and stage fright and drives away feelings of sorrow and discouragement, pessimism, lack of self-confidence, and lack of trust in others or of life in general. It also frees us from the need to remain absorbed by our problems. It develops intellectual abilities and improves perspicacity.

Eyebrow

Meridian: Urinary Bladder (paired with the Kidney meridian)

Element: Water

Emotional aim: Liberation from visceral fears and inhibitions that keep us from taking action. It resolves stagnation and frustrations. Develops inner strength and intuition, improves our emotional state, spurs ambition, and helps us develop the courage to make the necessary changes to get ourselves back on the "right track," the one that will allow us to fully express our innate talents.

Side of the Eye

Meridian: Gall Bladder (paired with the Liver meridian)

Element: Wood

Emotional aim: Freedom from feelings of rage, hatred, obsessive resentment, and the need for vengeance. Resolves feelings that are over the top and hectic. It helps the development of an accurate view of the whole of things and improves the constructive expression of anger. It also helps in the making of well-thought-out decisions, putting ideas into practice, and looking ahead with the strength of our past experience.

Under the Eye

Meridian: Stomach (paired with the Spleen-Pancreas meridian)

Element: Earth

Emotional aim: Freedom from excessive attachments, obsessional worries, and fixed notions. Resolves the emptiness we carry inside, deep dissatisfaction, and a lack of trust in the future. Develops the accurate expression of emotional feelings, improves good integration of experiences, opens the mind to new knowledge, helps in giving and receiving in a balanced way, and helps in feeling deeply satisfied.

Under the Nose

Meridian: Governor Channel (paired with the Functional Channel). Yang in nature, it is not connected with any element but governs the entire yang network of the meridians.

Emotional aim: Freedom from shyness, excessive modesty, and feeling ashamed of oneself, as well as from pathological self-control. It solves issues connected with clumsiness, difficulty revealing oneself to others, and the fear of speaking in public. This meridian develops personal character and originality, improves our ability to feel at ease in society, and gives us the audacity to live entirely independently of others' opinions, with no concern whatsoever for what others may think of us.

Hollow of the Chin

Meridian: Functional Channel (paired with the Governor Channel). Yin in nature, it is not connected to any element but rules the entire yin network of the meridians.

Emotional aim: Freedom from feelings of failure and guilt. Dispels regret and remorse; resolves feelings of depression and despondency, desolation, and torment. Improves the possibility of forgiving and forgetting. Offers relief from feeling the need to push down those who have done us wrong or the need to punish ourselves. Helps us accept things as they are and develop the will to forge ahead.

Collarbone

Meridian: Kidney (paired with the Urinary Bladder meridian)

Element: Water

Emotional aim: Freedom from the fears that prevent us from getting ahead in life and from living peacefully. Liberation from anxious neuroses and phobias (fear of solitude, crowds, heights, and so on). It reduces terror, agitation, and panic. Get into the habit of stimulating this point with the tips of your five fingers when you are submerged in a strong emotion (an urge to weep inappropriately, deep worry about someone, immense anger, panic, and so forth), and you will rapidly restore a sense of calm.

Under the Armpit

Meridian: Spleen-Pancreas (paired with the Stomach meridian)

Element: Earth

Emotional aim: Freedom from feelings that prevent us from fully incorporating the many joys of life. Reduces defeatist attitudes and feelings of pessimism, despondency, bitterness, boredom, and renunciation, as well as all ideas that repress pleasure and joy. Increases self-confidence and provides hope by strengthening sensations of contentment.

Under the Breast

Meridian: Liver (paired with the Gall Bladder meridian)

Element: Wood

Emotional aim: Freedom from distress, confusion, and inner vacillation. Reduces doubts, irresolution, and the narrow-mindedness that condemns us to stagnation and is a source of anger and frustration. Facilitates a healthy review of circumstances with a balanced evaluation of the facts. Helps us craft a plan of action, make important decisions, and bring about changes with full awareness.

Thumb

Meridian: Lung (paired with the Large Intestine meridian)

Element: Metal

Emotional aim: Freedom from profound afflictions and torments that turn into obsessions. Reduces inner suffering, susceptibility to misfortune, extreme sensitivities, and excessive generosity (in which the giver runs the risk of losing everything, including the self). Treats the internal wounds left by tragic events and emotional abuse.

Index Finger

Meridian: Large Intestine (paired with the Lung meridian)

Element: Metal

Emotional aim: Inner liberation by the absolution of offenses. Reduces the need to cling to grievances and sorrows and remain stuck in past misery. Eliminates rigidity of thought and the inflexibility of resentments. Facilitates a lenient attitude that will flourish once our interior wounds have been treated. It is a forgiveness that is also extended to ourselves, for all our past weaknesses and missteps.

Middle Finger

Meridian: Pericardium/circulation and sex (paired with the Triple Warmer meridian)

Element: Fire

Emotional aim: Freedom from feelings of inferiority

and lack of self-esteem. Frees us from the need to remain under the yoke of others. It facilitates the independence and free expression of our own personalities. It provides enthusiasm, excites passions while ensuring that they do not become excessive, and also treats problems connected with sexuality.

The ring finger is connected to the Triple Warmer meridian (paired with the Pericardium meridian), but it is left out of the complete EFT sequence because its function is identical to that of the Gamut point.

Little Finger

Meridian: Heart (paired with the Small Intestine meridian)

Element: Fire

Emotional aim: Freedom from the need to stay in the background as well as the necessity to hog the spotlight at any cost. For those who would do well to come out of their shells, to improve their finances, make friends, or find their "soul mate," the stimulation of this point diminishes fears connected to the wide world that supplies all our material and emotional resources.

The Gamut Point

Meridian: Triple Warmer (paired with the Pericardium meridian)

Element: Fire

Emotional aim: This point frees us from the imprisonment of our own certitudes. Stimulation of this point increases our ability to open our hearts (to give and receive affection and love) and reduces the need for isolation and withdrawal, which can lead to feeling rejected and abandoned by others. This point also soothes physical pain and depressive feelings.

6

The Various Ways
EFT Can Be Applied

STIMULATION OF THE POINTS
BY GENTLE PRESSURE

In some situations it is not necessary to actually tap on the meridian points to obtain excellent results. Gentle pressure on each point, while simultaneously taking a deep breath, is another frequently used method, and it allows EFT rounds to be performed in a more discreet manner. The sole difference lies in the longer time required for these sequences. Gentle pressure can, however, be a great substitute for tapping in the case of migraines or other physical discomfort.

IMAGINING STIMULATION OF THE POINTS

Once EFT has become a habit, you can also perform tapping rounds in your imagination. All you have to do is to close your eyes, concentrate on your problem, and mentally perform the sequences. This procedure works wonderfully if you are able to really focus your attention.

CONTINUOUS STIMULATION OF THE POINTS

When you feel as if you are drowning in a strong emotion, such as a panic attack, a fit of rage, or a strong desire to weep at an inopportune moment, you can skip the setup stage and go directly to the short tapping sequence, continuously stimulating the points from top to bottom, going back to the top to start the sequence again until you have recovered your calm.

STIMULATION OF A SINGLE POINT

For the same reasons, you can work on a single point until the emotion disappears completely. With experience you will note that there is one point in the sequence that seems to be particularly beneficial for you. Stimulate this favorite point, or that of the collarbone, when something upsets you, such as fear for someone close to you, an unpleasant thought, a painful memory, or a feeling of frustration, or when you keep dwelling on the same thoughts.

SIMULTANEOUS STIMULATION OF POINTS

Stimulation of the bilateral meridians can be performed on both sides simultaneously, if you like, or you can alternate between the two points. It may also be useful to tap the point beneath the nose and the one in the hollow spot of the chin at the same time.

EFT DURING NARRATION
OF A TRAUMATIC EPISODE

A common procedure in EFT practice is to perform a complete narration of a problem or tragic memory, with tapping applied judiciously along the way. This can be done alone or in the company of a friendly listener.

The story should begin *just before* the painful events took place and be relayed sequentially by recounting precisely what happened, coming to a complete stop when a painful emotion is triggered, in order to ensure performance of as many rounds as necessary to remove it completely.

If someone is present while you are narrating these events, it is recommended that the friend perform the tapping on your body whenever you are experiencing particularly difficult emotions. This will be of great help to you and ensure that the tapping continues without any interruption during this particularly trying passage.

You should then resume your story by repeating the example you just shared, which you should now be able to recount quite peacefully. If not, you must repeat the rounds until you are able to traverse this passage in a neutral fashion. The story is then continued until its conclusion, with immediate halts to apply EFT at the slightest sign of emotional disturbance. The event should then be repeated again in its entirety from start to finish, in order to ensure that no negative emotions that require treatment remain.

The story should be told in its most negative version possible with a maximum amount of emotion. Recount everything that passes through your mind. You can also speak while performing rounds continuously in both directions—going up from down and down from up while skipping the setup stage, unless you experience no relief to the pain. It is especially important to continue performing the rounds when you are going through violent emotions with tears, anger, or fright. Alternatively, you can stimulate a single point, which can be your favorite one, the Gamut point on the upper part of your hand, or the point on your collarbone. In this way you will be able to remove the energy blockages that are the true cause of all the torment you are experiencing.

If the story is particularly painful to recall, begin your rounds long before the tragic events with setups like these: "Even if this tragedy happened to me, I accept myself completely," or "Even if I am suffering intensely, I accept myself completely." You will then be able to approach these events, while in the process of performing your rounds, without having to undergo such intense suffering.

You should also never hesitate to perform EFT when other people are sharing their problems with you. If they are physically present, discreetly tap the Gamut point near the top of your hand, or apply strong pressure to the point by your collarbone with the tips of your five fingers. In other circumstances where no one can see you—for example, if you are on the phone—perform continuous rounds during the time the other person is speaking to you. You will be effectively helping that person on an energetic level while at the same time protecting yourself from his or her outpourings of painful emotions.

EFT FROM A DISTANCE

The practice of EFT over a distance makes it very clear that everything in our world is fundamentally connected. If you use it to try stopping a dog in the neighborhood from barking, or a child three rows back on an airplane from crying, you'll realize how much this is so. The results can be amazing.

EFT has two possible methods for performing treatment from a distance. You can either execute the tapping rounds on yourself, momentarily placing yourself in the place of the individual (or animal) you are seeking to treat, or you can imagine the stimulation of the tapping points on his or her body.

THE "EMERGENCY STOP" PROCEDURE

During times of high anxiety or panic attacks, the tapping sequence can be reduced to three points: the point under the eye, the point on the collarbone, and the point beneath the armpit. If you wish to do this discreetly, you can press each of these points while taking a deep breath rather than tapping.

TIME-SAVING SHORTCUTS

The short sequence takes only about twenty seconds, but other shortcuts are also possible. You can skip the setup stage, for example, and proceed directly to the round of tapping. Forty percent of the time we are not confronted by internal opposition, and the few seconds this saves can be precious. Resume doing the rounds preceded by the setup if you feel you are not making any progress.

Relief is also possible from carrying out the setup alone. Accepting your problem while stimulating the Sore Spot or the Karate Chop point is sometimes all that is needed to dispel a fear, a grievance, or a fit of anger.

ROLLING YOUR EYES
FROM FLOOR TO CEILING

To eliminate the little that remains of a painful emotion, rather than perform another round of tapping you can instead strike the Gamut point on the upper part of your hand while at the same time raising your eyes from the floor to the ceiling in a span of six seconds, while repeating the reminder of the problem to yourself.

ADDITIONAL POINTS

There are other frequently used points that can be helpful but are not part of the standard EFT sequence. These points can be found on the top of the head (toward the back), inside the wrist (at the place where a watch band is clasped), on the top of the wrist (at the placement of the face of the watch), and on the inside of the shin (where the fatty part of the calf begins).

VARIATIONS IN THE SETUP STAGE

The standard expression "I accept myself completely" takes into consideration the existence of a vast inner territory that dwells in the shadows, outside our waking consciousness. This consciousness consists of multiple fragments of the self at different ages that have been profoundly damaged by traumatic circumstances. When this happens the fragments no longer continue to grow or develop, but they don't just disappear. In truth, they are extremely active and find expression in all our problems.

The approval phrase that forms part of the setup serves to recover these fragmented parts of ourselves and wipe away the trouble they have caused as if with a sponge. This does not mean that we now find these troubles pleasant and invite them back for more. We simply stop hating and rejecting these immature aspects of our personality, each of which is only demanding a little bit of attention in its own way before rejoining the ranks.

The expression "I accept myself completely" signifies that we are abandoning our attempts to exclude them. In other words, we are accepting their separate existence. But it's possible to stipulate this consent in another way, if that has more appeal. For example, you could say, "Even if I lack affection, I recognize that a part of myself refuses to be nurtured, and I accept it completely."

You are thereby agreeing that a part of you feels unworthy of being loved, due to a variety of emotional abuses, and you take charge of it. The mechanism of taking ownership of the problem is then carried out completely naturally, with your subconscious mind creating the circumstances necessary for the healing of the emotional deficiencies in question.

7
EFT and the Realization of Goals

Each of us lives inside our own world, a world based on the belief systems that form our day-to-day reality. These beliefs are the fruits of our experiences and the conclusions we have drawn from them. The data of this personal perspective, stored inside our subconscious minds, is used to organize our lives.

This notion of the self controlling our reality is difficult to accept without raising an eyebrow. If we truly hold this power, we think, it is quite obvious that we would not intentionally use it to create problems for ourselves. We would use it in ways that would allow us to live healthy and fulfilled lives. This is simply one more conviction—a deceptive one, like so many others—that prevents us from taking the necessary steps to reach a state of deep contentment.

Everything we want and do not succeed in obtaining is held hostage by our subconscious mind. The barriers that confine us inside our difficulties are nothing but an amalgam of limiting beliefs. These narrow, utterly restrictive perceptions about our real possibilities are what EFT helps us change.

A difficult situation can be corrected by erasing its corresponding beliefs in the subconscious. Erroneous notions, despite the absolute value we may grant them, are prejudicial and toxic and arise uniquely from energy blockages anchored in our energy system. The path we follow with EFT allows us to free ourselves of them.

FIVE STEPS FOR CLEARING NEGATIVE THOUGHTS FROM THE SUBCONSCIOUS

The procedure is carried out in five stages that will erase the beliefs responsible and automatically leave a clear space for the positive convictions that reside just behind the limited ones. These are fruitful and progressive ideas that our limiting beliefs have repressed—limits founded on false conclusions about ourselves and the true nature of life.

The positive feelings that return can be summoned with a simple statement of the things we desire in life. This is usually all it takes for them to manifest concretely without any more difficulty.

First Stage

Write down the problem that is disturbing you most at this time—money troubles, difficulties at work, blemishes in your physical appearance . . . it does not matter as long as it is precise.

Second Stage

Present an exact description of what you would like to have in place of your problem. When you write it down, always begin your sentence with, for example, "I *have* a healthy body now," "I *am* successful in my career now," "I *feel* happy in my life now," and so on. Use terms that state that you already possess the thing you desire.

Third Stage

Emphatically state the preceding phrase (which should *precisely* describe the realization of your wish), and note in writing every negative thought that then enters your mind. The evocation of a lie of this nature should bring up lots of personal limiting beliefs. Empty your sack of objections to the very bottom, using as many pages as necessary. These are all the energy blockages that are forming an impenetrable barrier between your current situation and the one you would rather have in its place.

Fourth Stage

Out of your responses, select those that are the most wounding to you, or the most negative, and perform EFT sequences on each one specifically. If particular memories surface in your mind, erase their emotional impact immediately. Continue your cleansing session until you reach a point at which you can repeat your affirmation without causing negative feelings to arise. This will be a neutral position. You will not be experiencing great joy, but you will have the impression that all things are eventually possible.

Fifth Stage

Now proceed to "stating the positive" by tapping on the occipital bulge, the instructions for which can be found on page 49. It is during this stage that you will begin experiencing sensations of joy. This will produce a huge inner transformation of your beliefs, which will become the foundation for the betterment of your life henceforward in accordance with your desires.

THE UNWINDING PROCEDURE FOR THE REALIZATION OF FINANCIAL GOALS

Financial challenges are a common difficulty and cause of pain, so we will use financial hardship in an example of unwinding the objections and limiting beliefs that get in our way. When we eliminate these beliefs we release stuck energy that is blocking our growth and success.

1. **The problem:** A lack of income that is causing hardship and seems to be unending.
2. **The desired outcome:** "I am now living in great financial ease with large returns of money that come in stable and regular payments."

3. **The negative feelings (choose whichever apply):** "I do not have the abilities I need to earn money, my education is too limited, I am trapped in poverty forever, no one has ever helped me, I have too many responsibilities to think of finding a new job, it was a mistake to get married, I always go from one setback to another," and so on.

4. **The EFT sequences:** "I completely accept myself, even if I do not have the ability to earn money (reminder: inability to earn money), I completely accept myself, even if I am trapped in this poverty forever (reminder: trapped in this poverty)," and so on.

5. **The assertion of the positive (by tapping on the occipital bulge):** "I now enjoy complete financial security, I now have the means to easily obtain everything I need, the money I take in is now far more than my expenses, I now have a job that pays quite well, my life is now changing beyond my wildest expectations," and so on.

There are many possible ways to pull yourself out of a difficult situation, but they simply remain inaccessible as long as your subconscious mind remains opposed to your desire. Have you ever noticed how people are continually dealing with the same problems? They seem to be specializing in particular worries that follow them everywhere. And if there is an intermission now and then, the play resumes with an even more intense litany of similar worries.

This is only because the interior data remain unaltered.

Get rid of all these "yes buts" that you inevitably add on whenever you express one of your desires. You would like to begin painting, *yes, but* . . . you do not have the time, *yes, but* . . . you are not sure if you have talent, *yes, but* . . . being an artist means starving in a garret. Or you would like to change apartments, *yes, but* . . . the one you want is impossible to find. These are often accompanied by the most biased kinds of "yes buts" when they are turned back against you, statements such as *yes, but* . . . I am too ugly . . . too old . . . too broke . . . inferior to others . . . and so on. You are guaranteed to find proof for any of them in your current life.

Eliminate these negative responses as soon as they cross your mind. Bulldoze them away with EFT. They are nothing but horrible lies about your true possibilities. They are energy blockages anchored in your energy system and are easy to dissolve.

The deep-rooted ideas that are responsible for our problems cannot simply be undone by positive thinking alone, as some people try to make us believe. The subconscious cannot ever be duped, and this is why the practice of writing affirmations does not transform material reality. On their own, affirmations can actually amplify our problems.

The assiduous repetition of a phrase such as "I am financially prosperous," when everything is demonstrating to us the exact opposite, only serves to better anchor the contradiction. To eliminate a problem, we need to target it by dissolving the energy blockages that are responsible for it. Dissolving them one by one shows determination and persistence, the only skills required to work with EFT, which is otherwise easy to use and extremely effective.

Once you have altered the elements that are at the source of your problems, expect some surprises. Circumstances will work together to pull you out of your predicament. Things you never thought about will come to you. Unexpected encounters will occur. You will receive all the help you need.

8

Group Sessions
with EFT

Borrowing Benefits

The term *borrowing benefits* comes from the discovery of a healing connection that exists among all the participants in an EFT session, even though each individual is bringing a different problem to it. This borrowed ingredient offers considerable advantages. It makes it possible to enjoy EFT videos of different cases and is beneficial for small groups in which each individual in turn works on a problem in sessions that are useful to everyone.

These borrowing sessions are organized in accordance with a plan that produces the best results. For starters, it is quite specific. We already know that EFT must target a specific problem in order to be effective. This is an essential point, as we have a natural tendency to remain vague.

We express our problems in an overly general way with phrases such as "I am always out of money," "I am scared of being alone," or "Nobody loves me." But the real problem is elsewhere. It comes from specific emotional elements that have not yet been resolved and, for this reason, have provided the foundation for your problem. Indeed, how could a person say she was constantly hurting for money if that hardship were not evidenced by specific events? How can a person say he is frightened of solitude if he has not experienced the fear that can await us when we are alone? It is therefore necessary to discover which specific events formed the armature of our problems. The first place to look is in our memories.

WHAT DOES THIS PROBLEM BRING TO MIND?

The memories that surface, from the newest to the older ones, are the elements feeding our problems. But earlier we talked about the generalization effect, a natural shortcut that sweeps away the problem by removing the emotional charge connected to only some of these specific memories (from five to twenty is the current margin).

A situation that extended for several days, or even one that lasted only five minutes, is composed of segments that can be treated separately. A specific event, such as a stinging reply or a perverse glance, may have lasted only a few seconds. A permanent command given to the subconscious mind often depends on only a few details, and the deeper you go into the details of a situation, the better chance you will have of entirely eliminating the problem.

THE UNREELING
OF A GROUP SESSION

Each participant notes on a piece of paper the specific and precise incident to be treated, accompanied by a number from 0 to 10 that indicates the degree of its emotional intensity. For example, if you are afflicted by a fear of heights, do not write "my fear of heights," but rather, write "my panic on the mountain road when crossing the Alps," or "my terror at the idea that I was going to leap off the balcony," or "when that creep pushed me toward the edge of the cliff." The leader of the EFT session can also note a personal problem before starting.

While the EFT session is unfolding, each participant should repeat exactly the same words and stimulate the same points as the person for whom the treatment is being performed, while also casting a glance from time to time at his or her own personal problem. The person for whom the treatment is being performed reevaluates his or her level of suffering at the end of the session, which is frequently accompanied by surprise at finding the problem entirely resolved emotionally. If it is not resolved, it is fine to continue on the same problem during the following sessions. However, it is important to completely eliminate the emotional charge connected to the event being treated before passing on to the next individual's problem. All participants should check in with their own level of suffering at the end of each session as well, as participation in the group session can have a remarkably positive effect on everyone present.

It's possible that someone treating a problem in the presence of others will not verbalize it aloud, in which case the setup will take into account the discretion the individual wishes. The sentence will be spoken as "I accept myself completely, even though I have this problem," rather than going into detail. The evaluation of the level of suffering can then be used for the following setups, such as, for example, "I accept myself completely, even though my problem remains at level 8." The individual will concentrate strongly on the specific emotions being experienced, one at a time per round, as these are different aspects of the same problem. These can include shame, feelings of guilt, consequences of the problem, and so on.

9

Two EFT Variations

THE CHOICE METHOD

A much-used variation in EFT practice was conceived by Dr. Patricia Carrington. She calls it the Choice Method. The procedure is performed in a series of three successive rounds, equipped with a setup embellished with a positive choice. This is introduced as a substitute for the standard EFT phrase, "I accept myself completely," and comes directly after the problem has been declared, precisely expressing the desired alternative.

Good designation of the choice is essential here and requires a bit of skill. Many people are capable of describing their problem in great detail but are rendered speechless when they try to clearly express what they would like to have in its place. Obliged as we are when choosing this method to select a positive alternative, we find ourselves grasping for ideas.

With the Choice Method, a natural mechanism is set into motion in which every time the individual thinks about his or her problem, he or she also hears the preferred alternative. This will produce the desired attitude or changes, often with great rapidity.

Here is a detailed description of the method for a specific problem: "Even though I do not have enough insurance to pay for these water damages, I choose to find the means of making the repairs without any expense on my part, and I will be fully satisfied with the results."

The procedure opens by an evaluation of the level of the distress felt when evoking the problem, followed by the setup stage, stimulating the Sore Spot or the Karate Chop point, while repeating the phrase expressing the problem three times in a row, followed by the chosen solution, which will be our example: "Even though I do not have enough insurance to pay for these water damages, I choose to find a way to make the repairs without any expense on my part, and I will be fully satisfied with the results."

First Round

This round is performed while using only the reminder phrase of the problem at each point of the standard EFT sequence. Eyebrow: "these damages." Edge of the eye: "these damages," and so on.

Second Round

This round is performed immediately on the heels of the first (without any reevaluation of the distress level) while using only the reminder phrase of your chosen alternative. Eyebrow: "The repairs will be made without any expense on my part, and I will be fully satisfied with the results." Edge of the eye: "The repairs will be made without any expense on my part, and I will be fully satisfied with the results," and so on.

Third Round

This round is performed while alternately speaking the reminder of the problem and the positive option. Eyebrow: "these damages." Edge of the eye: "The repairs will be made without any expense on my part, and I will be fully satisfied with the results." Under the eye: "these damages," and so on, continuing to alternate and making sure to always end the round on the positive option. This will be the point beneath the breast when using the shortcut version and the Karate Chop point when using the long sequence (in which case, during the phase of the Gamut point, you will continue to introduce the reminder of the problem that was stipulated on the preceding point).

At this time there should be a new evaluation of your distress level, with a repetition of the three stages of this method, if called for, until the positive option emotionally becomes a possible alternative, with a little luck. And luck is precisely what we will receive once our inner blockages have been removed.

There is another variation, known as Emotional Freedom & Healing, which was created by Richard Ross, a highly regarded teacher and practitioner of energy healing modalities. The following exercise arose from his teaching and is a routine treatment that can cause profound changes when performed on a daily basis. The procedure works on the entire meridian network, incorporating a previously chosen phrase at each tapping point. It is intended to purify the entire energy system and does not require the targeting of specific problems as is necessary with EFT.

ROUTINE FOR THE CLEANSING
OF ENERGETIC BLOCKAGES

This procedure takes only several minutes, but it does call for a contemplative state in order to produce the desired inner transformation. It should be performed as a daily routine until positive changes are noticed.

Begin by taking some long, slow breaths in order to fully relax.

- **Sore Spot** (say the phrase three times in a row, preferably aloud, while massaging this point): "I accept myself completely, even though I have not yet been as successful in my life as I truly wish." Now maintain pressure on the point while taking a deep breath.
- **The Karate Chop point** (say the phrase three times in a row, preferably aloud, while tapping this point): "I now free myself from the deep elements that are hindering my development and the benefits necessary for my complete fulfillment." Now maintain pressure on this point while taking a deep breath.

Speak the following phrases only once at this time (preferably out loud), while tapping each point, then taking a deep breath after you have finished saying the phrase, maintaining pressure on the point.

- **Eyebrow:** "I easily free myself now from any deep-rooted elements that are still creating my ongoing feelings of adversity and suffering." Now maintain pressure on the point while taking a deep breath.
- **Edge of the eye:** "I easily free myself now from any deep-rooted elements that are still creating my ongoing states of hesitation and confusion." Now maintain pressure on the point while taking a deep breath.
- **Under the eye:** "I easily free myself now from any deep-rooted elements that are still creating my ongoing states of lack and hardship." Now maintain pressure on the point while taking a deep breath.
- **Under the nose:** "I easily free myself now from any deep-rooted elements that are still creating my ongoing states of powerlessness and resignation." Now maintain pressure on the point while taking a deep breath.
- **Hollow of the chin:** "I easily free myself now from any deep-rooted elements that are still causing my ongoing feelings of guilt and shame." Now maintain pressure on the point while taking a deep breath.
- **Collarbone:** "I easily free myself now from any deep-rooted elements that are still creating my ongoing states of fear and anxiety." Now maintain pressure on the point while taking a deep breath.
- **Under the armpit:** "I easily free myself now from any

deep-rooted elements that are still creating my ongoing states of sorrow and depression." Now maintain pressure on the point while taking a deep breath.

- **Under the breast:** "I easily free myself now from any deep-rooted elements that are still creating my ongoing states of anger and frustration." Now maintain pressure on the point while taking a deep breath.

- **On top of the head** (rest your hand flat on the top of your head and speak the phrase—preferably out loud): "I devote all the energy I have just recovered to the complete and easy unfolding of all my capacities for personal realization." Take a deep breath when you have finished saying this.

- **Tapping on the occipital bulge** (choose one or more phrases from the following list, or create your own affirmations based on your personal desires, and repeat them three times in a row, preferably out loud):

"Every day I discover more of the full range of my skills and I am now expressing myself fully."

"I am now becoming more and more aware of my countless talents and great qualities."

"My life is now becoming a source of deep satisfaction in every domain."

"I am amazed by all the great opportunities that are opening up to me."

"The changes I want are occurring in a pleasant and easy way."

"I am now receiving all the material and emotional support I need."

"My life is now transforming beyond my wildest dreams."

"New financial possibilities are now bringing me great material security."

"Joyful circumstances are now propelling me into a state of financial abundance."

"I now feel protected, loved, and respected."

"I am seeing things from a new angle now and it is bringing me profound tranquillity."

"I consent to feeling all the joy and happiness to which I am completely entitled."

"I am presently harvesting all the benefits that are due to me."

"My work is inspiring and quite lucrative."

"I know it is possible for me to greatly improve my life."

"I am spilling over with new ideas and the means to put them into practice."

"I clearly see what I want and I have the power to achieve all my ambitions."

"I follow my heart's enthusiasm and enact my plans as I wish them to be realized."

"I have the courage to carry out the transformations I wish to see happen."

"My life is now blossoming fully thanks to the techniques of Tapping!"

10
In Conclusion

EFT is like a crane that clears the plot of land on which you want to build your dream house. The only difference is that the house builds itself once the terrain has been cleared. This house represents your potential that has been buried beneath a mountain of limiting beliefs and false assumptions. Remove them and you will find a magnificent property with amazing features.

To prepare the ground you need only put EFT to work on everything that is holding you back from realizing your dreams. Whether there are bundles of twigs or enormous boulders, this brilliant tool will eliminate them for you. The bad memories that haunt you, the stress of daily life, and the fear of what the future might bring are all nothing but energy. They are simply a vaporous substance that the smallest puff of breath can chase away.

These new modalities of energy treatments are completely overturning our concepts of healing. Could a simple technique designed to balance the energy flow coursing through our bodies be the key to our well-being? It is up to you to discover. Test it at once on a fear, an old pain, or something that is tormenting you. One round of Tapping can be performed in less than a minute. It sometimes takes only one or two rounds to recover full serenity.

EFT and the other methods of this kind all share one point in common: they stimulate the energy system while the individual remains fully focused on the problem for which resolution is sought. It is therefore necessary to begin by accepting our emotions in all their negativity so that we can then rid ourselves of them. In other words, when we stop repressing and fighting against them, we'll find that our problems are not the real problem. The real difficulty is the emotions that remain trapped inside of us in the form of energy blockages. They are the undeniable reflection of fundamental needs that we refuse to consciously acknowledge.

To ensure that EFT works well, start by feeling the sadness and frustration that are the cause of all your hardships, down to your deepest place. Also accept the feelings of anger that arise when you think about all your deficiencies and failings. These feelings are indicative of energy blockages, and they are also responsible for the problems and disruptions that afflict you in your day-to-day life. They are the results of your restricted view of your own abilities, the abilities of others, and the general workings of the world. This perception is often tragic in nature as it is based on your experiences and has no other value than the one you grant it.

Take one negative feeling at a time—a fear, a bad memory, a fixed idea—and feel it disappear during the course of your EFT rounds. Use the language that best expresses your personal truth. This is no time to mind your manners. You must boldly enter the region of your greatest suffering and weakness. You will come out on the other side as shiny as a new penny.

Remember, EFT is a tool that will accompany you everywhere if you remember to use it. Use it when you are going through difficult times or to improve your performance in work or play. Do not allow anything to slip past you. EFT is extremely effective. You will be astonished at the easy transformation of your problems.

A PERSONAL NOTE

As a longtime specialist of feng shui, I discovered EFT when I was looking for ways to improve the effect of this ancient Chinese discipline. As you may be aware, feng shui is used to maintain balance and harmony in our homes so that the energy is conducive to well-being and prosperity, but I was not entirely convinced of its effectiveness. I was especially concerned by the irregularity of its effectiveness and could not understand the reason for this.

Yet it is not feng shui that should be called into question here, but that inner opposition that prevents things from running smoothly. Feng shui always provides excellent results when its precepts are observed. However, therein lies the problem. There are steps we just cannot take. It is not because they are expensive; they are often easy to implement with everything we need at hand. The problem is that there is something inside us that opposes them. This situation is made all the stranger by virtue of the fact that these steps are directly connected to the solution to our problems. What we are dealing with here is obviously that well-known psychological reversal, which, for obscure reasons, forces us to act contrary to our conscious wishes. This sneaky means of spoiling our lives can be easily treated with EFT.

I now combine EFT with my feng shui practice and teach it to my clients to hasten the arrival of what they desire. In other words, I use it to help them eliminate their own internal opposition. Of course, I also use it personally on myself when something upsetting occurs.

With EFT there is no longer any question that a fear, an unpleasant memory, or a poisonous thought is best handled by sternly lecturing yourself, which, as you know, doesn't work. The energetic disruptions that such negativities can create can be addressed immediately with EFT in more effective ways. Gone are all those feelings of guilt that latch on to negative thoughts when we have been soothing ourselves, sometimes even deluding ourselves, with "positive thinking" precepts. These precepts impose a practice in which we must always think in positive ways in order to allegedly manifest the life of our dreams.

It is certainly true that our limiting beliefs and utterly negative thoughts are responsible for all our problems, but it is never by repressing them, or flipping them like pancakes, that we can settle all our troubles. Our negative feelings are telling us something, and it is not a bad thing to lend them an ear. On the contrary, refusing to listen to what is going on inside is truly detrimental.

Emotions are nothing but the energy that is moving through our bodies. A free trajectory corresponds to a positive emotion, while an obstructed path corresponds to a painful or limited thought. In short, it involves a simple mechanism that we have no good reason to fear. This is all the more true since the advent of EFT, in which a snap of the fingers can restore the flow of the energy system.

A SESSION REPORT TAKEN
FROM GARY CRAIG'S INTERNET SITE

To bring this handbook to a beautiful conclusion, here is the gist of an account of a session led by Catherine O' Driscoll, an EFT practitioner in Scotland. I chose it because of its particularly interesting setup stage, which permitted, against all expectations, the resolution of a serious physical problem by unearthing its specific emotional cause. It is also a summary of the letter sent to EFT's creator, Gary Craig, the complete version of which can be found on his site.

◇◇◇

Glen is a true gentleman who came to me with his head hanging forward, in absolute pain. He had been wearing a neck collar for three months. His doctor had referred him to a specialist and the specialist had referred him to another specialist. A physiotherapist was involved. Eventually Glen took himself to a chiropractor. No one was sure what was wrong with him.

CAT scans were next. Glen's doctors hadn't seen anything like this before. The chiropractor said the closest description of his condition was a thing called "drop neck," which horses suffer. The physiotherapist consulted all her medical books and thought it might be a condition known as "dystonia," which is an incurable neurological condition. She suggested that surgery might be appropriate—an operation that is chancy at best. It could go horribly wrong.

Glen was terrified that he might have to stop working. He had no idea how he would pay his bills if this condition couldn't be cured, and he was terrified that he would never get better.

We tapped on this: . . . "even though I might never get better . . . even though I might not be able to work . . ."

Throughout the hour-long consultation, we measured Glen's neck pain on a 0 to 10 scale. It stayed up there at 10 throughout.

I knew darn well that Glen didn't have an incurable condition. To me, he was suffering from stress. I knew this because Glen is my brother-in-law, and I'd watched him cope with tremendous obstacles over the past few years. At last I had him in my treatment room—he lives in England and I live in Scotland—so I was determined to help Glen recover while he was visiting.

Here are just some of the obvious stress issues involved:

1. Glen and his wife (my sister) Leslie are great animal lovers. To them, their dogs are their children. Three of their dogs died last year, and their grief was huge.

2. Our father has been suffering from dementia for the last three years. He's been living in a home in England and my sisters and their husbands have been visiting him every day, staying for hours and coping with a man they remember as someone very special, but who is now throwing furniture at them and raving, or crying, or singing, or pacing up and down. They've been going through terrible emotional turmoil, watching my father suffer.

3. Leslie and Glen have also been coping with Glen's mother, who also has dementia, and her sister, who has had several strokes. Glen and Les had to fly to Ireland and attend to their affairs, selling the family home and auctioning off their possessions to pay for nursing care. Glen has been traveling to and from Ireland every two months to attend to his mother's and aunt's needs. This means that Glen has no vacation time left.

4. And then Leslie came down with clinical depression, leaving Glen to bear the burden of it all. She's getting better now—but that's another EFT story.

So Glen and I sat in my treatment room and discussed all that had been happening. I asked him if he felt that life was a bit of a burden and if he sometimes resented what was happening. I asked if he felt unsupported. "No," he said. "I'm just glad I'm there to help my mother. I'm glad I can help Les through her depression. It's great to be there for your dad."

Now, it comes in handy sometimes to be a selfish sort of a person—someone (like me) who would moan like mad if I had all the responsibilities Glen had. It didn't make sense to me that Glen didn't mind even just a little bit. He told me that he had had a fabulous childhood. He said he really felt a lot of guilt about joining the RAF and gadding about, leaving his mum alone when he was a young man. He was glad to make it up to her now.

We tapped on all sorts of things relating to Glen's neck pain—the pain itself, the fear surrounding the pain, the incurable diagnosis. The pain level stayed at 10.

And then, almost despairing, I decided to go for broke. Tapping his Karate Chop point, Glen repeated after me (whether he agreed or resonated with what I was asking him to say or not): "Even though I have this incurable neck pain . . . And even though I let my mum down when I was younger . . . I love myself . . . I'm okay . . . And even though life is a tremendous burden . . . And life is a pain in the neck . . . And I can't fix everything for everyone . . . And I can't stop people suffering . . . I'm okay. I accept myself. And even though I can't cope with everything and I feel unsupported . . . I matter . . . And I thank my body for giving me this gift . . . For telling me I have to stop and think of me, too . . . And even though I can't fix everything . . . I'm a good boy." At which point Glen burst out laughing and his neck pain lifted. We walked into the garden giggling like little children, with sparks of light flying around us.

The next day Glen had no more need of his neck collar.

He and Leslie tapped again last night, and Glen felt further relief. He knows now that he will be able to continue working. He knows there's no need for a dangerous operation. He knows that his body was giving him a precious gift—the knowledge that he also has to be on his list of people who matter. Like Leslie's depression, Glen's body was saying, "Enough!" It made him listen.

I shudder to think what would have happened to Glen had EFT not been there for him. He won't stop helping his loved ones, but he's going to start helping himself as well.

WHO IS AUTHORIZED TO USE EFT?

Although EFT is used by many health professionals in both the physical and mental health fields, the technique belongs to everyone. Anybody can use it with the stipulation that they do not call themselves therapists unless they are already accredited in that profession. No harmful effect has ever been observed in the use of EFT. There may be slight fatigue due to relaxation, or sometimes violent weeping that is quickly relieved by tapping, but that is pretty much all.

Gary Craig offers an enormous manual for free on the extremely extensive website he created to teach EFT (www .emofree.com) and encourages people to make full use of all his material with no request for permission, so long as the material is used ethically.

Resources

ONLINE RESOURCES

There is a wealth of information on EFT and other modalities of energy psychology and energy medicine on the Internet. I have listed some recommended resources in alphabetical order below.

Association for Comprehensive Energy Psychology (ACEP)
www.energypsych.org
ACEP is an international resource and networking tool offering workshops, training, and certification in EFT and other mind-body techniques.

Gary Craig
www.emofree.com
Gary Craig, who originated EFT (Emotional Freedom Technique), hosts this website offering his free manual and an abundance of supporting literature, including a vast selection of CDs and videos for learning EFT at little or no cost. Also available: free advanced video sessions and a subscription to his weekly newsletter.

Danielle Duperret, N.D., Ph.D.
danielleduperret.com

Dr. Duperret, a practitioner of energy medicine, is a doctor of naturopathy with a Ph.D. in natural health. She offers a free "discovery session" via her website and works with clients around the world via Skype in either English or French.

EFT Support Groups
www.groups.yahoo.com, www.meetup.com

It can be helpful to meet locally with others who have used the protocol or are simply curious about the process.

David Feinstein, Ph.D.
www.innersource.net

Dr. Feinstein, a clinical psychologist, is an internationally recognized leader in the rapidly emerging field of energy psychology. His website includes a good interactive map that lists EFT practitioners with descriptive bios from all over the country.

Fred Gallo, Ph.D.
www.energypsych.com

Dr. Gallo is a luminary in the field of energy psychology. He developed advanced energy psychology (AEP) and offers training and certification in a number of different countries. His entire website allows the user to choose from dozens of different languages and offers links to practitioners around the world.

Sophie Merle
www.SophieMerle.com

Sophie Merle, the author of this book, directs an extensive website (in French), which she established to promote the benefits of EFT and other energy healing modalities in the French-speaking countries of the world.

John Newton
www.healthbeyondbelief.com
John Newton is not strictly an EFT practitioner, although he includes the protocol in his work. He offers a series of sessions in Ancestral Clearing to clear the unresolved burden of events that have happened to our ancestors in the past, often referred to as "karma."

Brad Yates
www.bradyates.net
Brad is known internationally for his creative and often humorous use of EFT. A certified hypnotherapist, he combines this background with training in energy psychology and techniques for personal growth and achievement. He coaches groups and individuals in achieving greater success, health, and happiness. He offers monthly live teleseminars and has posted more than 200 instructional videos on YouTube.

RECOMMENDED READING

Numerous books have been written on various aspects of energy psychology and related fields. These are some of the most noteworthy.

EFT

Energy Tapping: How to Rapidly Eliminate Anxiety, Depression, Cravings, and More Using Energy Psychology, by Fred Gallo, Ph.D. (New Harbinger Publications, 2008, 2nd ed.).

The Promise of Energy Psychology: Revolutionary Tools for Dramatic Personal Change, by David Feinstein (Jeremy P. Tarcher/ Penguin Group, 2005, 3rd ed.).

Neuroscience

The Biology of Belief: Unleashing the Power of Consciousness, Matter & Miracles, by Bruce Lipton, Ph.D. (Hay House, 2008, rev. ed.).

Quantum Physics

Eye to Eye: Quest for the New Paradigm, by Ken Wilber (Shambhala, 2001, 3rd ed.).

The Field: The Quest for the Secret Force of the Universe, by Lynne McTaggart (HarperCollins, 2002).

The God Particle: If the Universe Is the Answer, What Is the Question?, by Leon Lederman and Dick Teresi (Houghton Mifflin, 1993).

Index